TESTAMENT

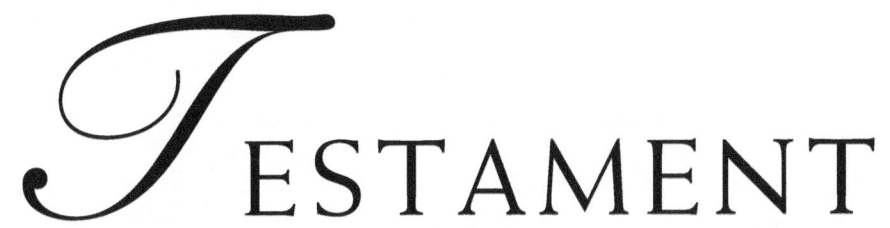

TESTAMENT

*My Survival and Conquest
of Breast Cancer*

ROBIN DYE

iUniverse, Inc.
New York Lincoln Shanghai

Testament
My Survival and Conquest of Breast Cancer

iUniverse books may be ordered through booksellers or by contacting:

iUniverse
2021 Pine Lake Road, Suite 100
Lincoln, NE 68512
www.iuniverse.com
1-800-Authors (1-800-288-4677)

Because of the dynamic nature of the Internet, any Web addresses or links contained in this book may have changed since publication and may no longer be valid.

ISBN: 978-0-595-40820-7 (pbk)
ISBN: 978-0-595-85183-6 (ebk)

Printed in the United States of America

God. Mine, yours and our; God is truly, without pause or hesitation, my reason for Testament. In my opinion, and His, our Lord is your reason to witness.

True friends. I mean, "true" friends. How very rare they are. That's why I dedicate my book and my survival/conquers to my God, who had the foresight to give me a strong spirit and a sense of humor, and my true friends. My "best" and "true" friend is Cheryl Peacock. Who always pushes me to be my inner self's' best. Especially, when I don't want to be and I feel like letting myself, and the heavy load down. Jonathan or to me, Jon who if I may have Jehovah's' blessing will be my eternal partner. I also must dedicate it to my father, who has given me "me". Made me who I am, with his knowledge, love and "never die" attitude. I dedicate to Jim, who is my true human "guardian". Then there is, of course, my "Jo". Dr. Joseph Kingsbury. He is the only man; whether he is a doctor or not, who has, honestly, seen me "inside and out". I couldn't have made it without my Jehovah, all my loved ones, and all the others who made me strong through them. Thanks to you for carrying me when I was too weak to walk. Bless you all. Oh wait; He already, did.

Contents

Acknowledgements . . . . *ix*

Me~Robin Renee. . . . . *xi*

The Day. 1

Diagnosis 3

Doctors 5

Clarity 9

Fear 13

3 days. 72 hours 15

Vivid 17

Oh God … help us. 19

The Hunt: 23

Dr. Kingsbury and his "Plan To Fight" .25

CHEMO-Therapy 27

Picking out the boob 29

The eyelash 31

The Sick Days 33

Memories~ 35

Friends 37

Off with the wig! 41

~ Reflect ~ 43

Final Thought~ 45

Acknowledgements

"New World Translation of The Holy Scriptures" 1984 Edition published by the Watch Tower Bible and Tract Society of New York, Incorporated.

"Women's Devotional Bible" New International Version 1980 Edition published by the Zondervan Publishing House in 1980.

"The Kingdom Interlinear Translation of the Greek Scriptures" 1985 Copyright by Watch Tower Bible and Tract Society of Pennsylvania and International Bible Students Association.

"The NIV Study Bible" 1985 Edition published by Zondervan Bible Publishers Grand Rapids, Michigan 49506,USA

Me~Robin Renee

Who am I? Where do I start? Writing this book now; 7 years, and a couple other "traumas" later, knowing what the last chapter of this book is going to be, well, is kind of like acting surprised at what you got for Christmas; even so you and your 4 brothers and sisters steamed opened every single present, put them back in the closet in perfect locations, and already know. We still acted amazed, though.

Every advisor, editor, friend and, of course, Cheryl suggest; a little too strongly mind you, that I give some insight as to who I am, or who I was before all the traumas or before the "dramas, after the traumas". I am suppose to tell you about the woman that got murdered in the story, before she gets shot, so you, the reader, has empathy for her. Hum. I don't want sympathy, or empathy, for that matter. I do, however, regrettably, see their point. Man, I dislike that, strongly. Not being able to do anything, other than stall, and stare at the curser on a blank Microsoft file for the last day, I have decided, enough of that. Write on.

I am, or I was at the start of this, a 30 year old female, of true, and proud Latin/Portuguese decent. I was, and am still Robin Renee Lemos Raya Dye.

I have an above average radio sales job, with an above average financial income, and the husband with a beautiful daughter and house to match.

I am one of 6 children, 5 of which were truly significant in my life. There is my fathers' first son, from his first wife; he's only had like … um 6 wives, but we don't acknowledge that son, as part of our "family unit".

I believe that to be his choice, the son, and when my father asks me, "Out of respect for him" being my father, to drop the whole issue. Oh yeah, it's dropped; like a "cow peeing on a flat rock". That's a dad term. I digress, again. My father was a Master Gunnies Sergeant in the Marine Corp, with some time in as a drill SSgt. Mix that in with the whole "Proud Portuguese" deal, and to say he was "strict" would be like asking "does a crack head crave a ten dollar "pebble"? *Yeah.* I start by telling you who I am, by telling, who he is. My father is a very big piece of my own puzzle. He has molded, the puzzle of, me. I am so proud to be his daughter. Do yourself a favor, appreciate your family, don't judge them, I think that's' on HIS "LIST". Because, we've truly, never walked in someone else's shoes. We may have the same style shoe, or the color, but not "that" shoe, not exactly. It was a very hard thing for me to learn, and to continue to do.

Matthew 7:1,2.Do not judge, or you too will be judged. For in the same way you judge others, you will be judged, and with the measure you use, it will be measured to you.

The Day

The day. What a day, but in the end, it was just like the stories read, it was just like any other day. Morning was breaking, the sun was rising and I was lying in bed, caressing myself. My chest. I was caressing my swollen tummy, with my baby inside. Comfortingly. Like your mom caresses your hair when you're a child. Then unexpectedly, I felt it, what felt like a walnut in my right breast. Odd enough it sort of carried over to my armpit. With more of it in my armpit, so this caused me no alarm what so ever. You can't have breast cancer in your armpit, right? Besides I have had fibro-cystic, the disease that causes lumps in your breast during and after your cycle, since I was a teenager so this was no big deal to me. At a very young age, I started having my yummy breast, or at least I thought, and think they were, looked at by barf green, hospital gowned, doctors. What's another doctor or lump for that matter? If only for a split second, though I let my mind think, what if? What if this was "cancer"? And then as quickly as I thought, "what if" came into my mind I pushed the thought aside. That would be the ultimate bad joke, huh?

No way, someone like myself, Robin Renee, at the top of my game professionally and parentally, who's getting ready to decorate my new babies' room, in my bran new house ... would get cancer, no way. I refuse it to be. I absolutely refused it. No. I would not allow it.

In the end, cancer doesn't care what the heck *you* refuse, or even who *you* are. It, like most diseases is non-prejudicial. It tries to bring down any color, any race, any religion, and any sex. The bastards. I have learned, and what you must also, is that you must decide in your mind, not to let it win. Like going up against the toughest sports competitor. You have to determine, if only in your own mind and heart, that you're going to win. Period. It doesn't matter the odds, the chances, and prognosis. You must make yourself win. You may still lose the fight or the game by twenty but you will lose with honor in not being a loser. A loser to me is someone, anyone that gives up.

Especially if it is your own self you're selling short. Don't do it. Don't, for the love of God, and all that it right in your life and world, give up on you! Ever. Period. Never. *You never, ever, never give up, on you!*

Psalm55: 22 Cast your cares on the Lord and he will sustain you; he will never let the righteous fall.

Diagnosis

My husband. What a huge pain in the ass he can be. I mean why is he so hard on me about this stupid lump in my breast? Give me a break. Hello … I'm six months pregnant. Honey, at this point, I've got lumps everywhere. And not just lumps either. I'm sure if I was brave enough to look at myself in the mirror naked I'd find I'm carrying the whole Ben and Jerry's' frozen dessert section in chunks on my lower extremities, starting with my rear. But he is, and so I'm here. Sitting. Waiting.

I was waiting outside my gynos' office in a reception area filled with more "Parent" magazines and maternity catalogs than you could ever imagine. Waiting, like all the others, with one thing in common. We're either pregnant, trying to be, or just were; or we've all got to pee! But you know you have to wait to get called back and do the whole sample thing. So you wait, and try to smile, while you're all about to float away from the two ice teas you had at lunchtime. Being pregnant … they weren't the "long Island" type of teas either.

Great! It's my turn. I vote to do the pee sample prior to the weigh in. The first reason is obvious the second is my hope it will drop me a pound or two and it will justify a stop at 31 flavors on the way home. And even so these are suppose to be the best Drs.' in town, I still find it kind of offensive that they rotate you around between seven doc-tors like some form of cattle call.

They say that they never know "who will be on call the night you have your baby, and they want you to recognize all of the seven faces" that might be looking up at you from your crotch. Okay, they don't put it exactly like that, but that's what it boils down to. What really gets to me is it means I only get to see the cute one once every sev-enth visit. That's not today, either. Blast. Shoot. Crap.

Doctors

Going through a lengthy medical condition you learn several things about Docs. Not only do doctors vary in their looks, ranging from "drop dead" (pardon the expression) gorgeous ... to "one breath from death" butt ugly.

But also amazingly even so they all went through the same schooling system and studied the same books; they differ in everything from bedside mannerism to actual prognosis. For the patient, it's pretty much a crapshoot at best. They know it, that's why *they* created second opinions. Either that or they are giving each other kickback for referrals. In the end it boils down to this ... It is a customer service they are providing. And *you* are the customer. You keep asking, pushing, demanding, testing, and going back until you are satisfied. Or, you find someone else. *Period.* I have seen more doctors than I hope you can imagine. I have yet to see any one of them walk on water. Can you "Dig it"? The first step, in any struggle w/the medical community is to lay down the law as to how you expect your care to proceed. Demand high respect and aggressiveness and they will follow. I made it clear that only this wrapped around/a positive attitude was tolerable. With that, back to the doctor's office I go. I'm sure that the only one thing that surpasses *this* doctors' intelligence; is his *arrogance.* He is, in general opinion, "the best of the group" as far as experience and skill *but bedside manner?* The sisters in catholic school had a better demeanor. That's okay though because it will be brief and painless. He's going to tell me the same thing that every other doctor has told me in the past. It's a cyst. If you want it out ... we'll take it out. If you want to leave it in, then leave it in. Being the careful one, I've always opted for taking it out. Of course, that's also why at the ripe age of thirty my breasts look like they done a couple tours in war torn countries, or had rough some pretty rough sexual partners. For the sake of my mom, and hopefully, a lot of the "general public" who's going to read this book, it wasn't the later. Just an option they give you.

Those weren't the options he gave me though. He didn't give an option, if I remember correctly. I'm not sure. Looking back, some events are very clear, yet others, I'm sure I must have went into some sort of shock because I am sure it happened, I just don't remember. I mean, I can remember being there. I just can't lay it out in detailed form. There are only big huge blocks of time. Other times, it's as if it *just* happened it's so clear.

The funny thing, (Not funny like ha-ha, piss your pants funny but funny like "hmm", like Arsenal Hall use to do in his show) is that there does not seem to be any rhyme or reason in my brains selection. They say that it is your brains way of protecting you. It puts it all deep inside you're subconscious, and sends you on your way. Which is okay and good until one sunny day for no apparent reason, some stupid country song has you pulling over, in the middle of your day, on the freeway. You sob uncontrollably for hours upon hours.

Listen, seriously, my suggestion, if you are currently going through any real trial in you life, what you feel is a "Godforsaken" period, or test/trial ... leaving the country stations alone. He felt it. The little lump that is no bigger than a grape. I watched him. I watched his eyes. My father, being a true Latin Portuguese, gave me that lesson a long time ago. If you want to learn the "truth", or what they think the "truth" is to them, look at their eyes. People can control how they *"act"* and what they say. *"Reaction"*. Now, that is what holds the truth. It's like coming around the aisle of your comfortable, local grocery store and someone from high school that you haven't seen in years is boom, right there. And they're in a ... wheelchair. The first look, that's brutal truth. That's reaction.

His *reaction*, made me very uneasy. But, what came out of his mouth was smooth, and calm. Especially for Mr. No Couth. "I can't conclude by palpitation, have to send you to an associate, blah, blah, blah ..." Of course, the fact that he called him, was sending me over to see this associate/surgeon right away, should be telling me something. It should of told, right then. Oh course, no, not me.

Now, either I drove over to the surgeon, or Jesus, but one of us got me there. After peeing and leaving the gyno's office I don't remember anything at all. Not getting in the car, not driving, not parking. So, what's that tell you? I try to see the "action", and not get fooled by "reactions". Try being the key word here.

Galatians 6:4.Each one should test his own actions. Then he can take pride in himself without comparing himself to somebody else, for each one should carry his own load.

Clarity

Here is where it gets clearer, though. At that moment, I snapped. Right there, in the surgeons office. I knew. I knew that I had cancer. Before he examined me, before the grave look of concerned reaction, before he called radiology and told them "he was sending me down right now and for them to fit me in right away", oh yeah, I knew. But I wasn't scared! Not, yet. I was in control. If I just stay calm and in control, this will all go away. I'm just going to be pissed for these people wasting my whole day. I waited for the ultrasound he sent me for. The first one I had on my breast, and not my pregnant stomach. I was scheduled to have the babies' final ultrasound in one week. I was thinking of that for a long time during the whole process of cold jelly and the rolling of the machinery across my breast. Laying there it also occurs to me just how may people get the "distinct privilege" of looking at *my* breasts. I'm sure that's why my brother is a doctor. Face it people! Unless you're a *proctologist* your day is pretty damn sweet. At some time during the day, you're going to see someone naked. Beats the hell out of selling radio, or getting paid to make "sub sandwiches" a day, I'll tell you that.

I waited for the radiologist to give me my films. I walked to the phone and placed only one call. Only one. My husband? No. My mom? My father? No. Brothers? Sisters? Second cousins/twice removed? *No!* My boss. Isn't that weird? I called her to tell her I didn't think I would be making it back to work today because they wanted to do some tests. I felt bad for skipping the day because I'd only been there a week when I found out I was pregnant in the first place. Little did either one of us know that this one phone call would mark the beginning of the deepest friendship I've ever known. One tested, strengthened, and cherished and adored. How calm I was. I remember telling myself over and over, I'm in control, and I'm in control. I remember telling myself, was over and over, and over again. I am so completely in control.

Then I walked to the bathroom, opened the stall and, calmly barfed my brains out and half my stomach. Okay. I'm in control. I'm in control. Over and over … Back up the elevator I go with films in hand. Yep, *"surgery is a must"* to determine what it is. "Please come back tomorrow with your husband and we'll discuss it all". This is what Mr. Couth had to say. I feel confident in this mans/Dr.s' hand. He is older and appears distinguished. He has an air about him that is kind of hard for me to explain. He strikes me like a Ricardo Montalban or my Dad in his "Hey Day." He seems intense, but he wasn't running around "summoning the Gods"(which I was sure they did if someone had the "c" word). What is left to do? I went home. Thank God, Jesus wasn't busy, because I am, absolutely sure, he drove again. Telling Jim.

You would think that *it* would stand out in my mind. To tell your newlywed husband, the man whose been by your side for five years, the father of your unborn child you "might" have cancer.

But honestly, I can't remember how, or even when. There is no such conversation or facial image in my mind. I'm sure it must have been that night because he would have been on me about what happened at the obgyn office.

Not to mention I had to look like an "Alice Cooper Groupie" by the time I got home. But I don't remember, I pray, I never do. The facial image must have been heart breaking, beyond words.

Seven months ago we watched as his mothers ashes were scattered on the ocean in burial.

They say she died of "breast" cancer. I'm sure it was the "chemo" that killed her. I swore to him, right then that "when" I got cancer, I would rather die than have chemo. We won't even talk about taking my breast. No way. Not me. I'd rather die. And when I say "when" I get cancer it's because I knew I would. Somehow, I knew. When he used to get on me about my driving, as all "men" do, I've realized; I would say, "Don't worry, I'm not going to die in the car. I'm going to die of cancer". Right about then, I felt like a total ass.

I never *know* what I will do in a "burning building" … I haven't been in one. Do you *know* what you will do?

Corinthians 8:1 .We know we all possess knowledge. Knowledge puffs up but love builds up. The man who thinks he knows something does not yet know, as he ought to know.

Fear

The fear of God must have come into Jims' mind. I do not know if possible, worse than me. Imagine that one.

I was in absolute control. I wasn't worried. Even so I knew, deep down in my very core, I knew. I had it. Nothing was concrete though, until they tell me, face to face.

In the "Ricardo Montalban"/surgeons' office, I'm certain we asked a lot of questions. None of which either stand out in my mind, now, or really seemed to have a chance to change anything.

They "have to have it in their hands" to tell you. Everything up to that point is "mere speculation". The main focus for me was the baby. Six months pregnant. Facing a lumpectomy. Of course, I had had lumpectomies prior to this day. I had had six lumpectomies, prior to this one. But this one is not the same. I knew. The surgeon we had at the time decided to do the lumpectomy under locale anesthesia. I would not be asleep at all, which was the best thing for the baby in his eyes. Of course, I hadn't slept in three days anyway, so what the heck, what are another 3? Okay … where do I sign? When do we start? Let's do it right now.

3 days. 72 hours

It was to prove to be the longest stretch of time I had ever experienced in my life. Inside I was mush. Outside? Outside? I was in control. A rock. I went to work; I kept a smile, and acted as though it was just another day. Only Jim, close family, and my best friend really "knew". I didn't want anyone else to know because you see; I'm the funny one. By that I mean I am the upbeat one. The one with all the jokes is I. The one who brings you up when you are down. And I wasn't ready or willing to be on the other side of that coin. I'm still not. I fully believe that we are not the people we are because of the dish life gave us. Not because of our skin, or our looks, although I thank God daily I'm not ugly … just vain! Ha!

But seriously, it is our attitude and sense of life that makes us who we are. It will inevitably determine our fate. Believing this is what got me through those few days, and the many to come. My hope is that if you are going through some form of personal hell, even if its just "life", it will help you too. Events happen … good and bad, to good and bad people. What you do from there; that is what determines, who you are.

Eccl 9:11 Time and unforeseen occurrence befall them all

It's time. Sitting on the edge of the hospital bed, it seemed like the edge of life for that matter, I am amazingly calm. Calm to everyone, but only calm on the outside. Jim and I kind of tiptoed around the issue up till this point. Almost as if talking about it, would some how give it some type of validity? When we did talk, it was clean cut. Just the facts, ma'am. As if we had a mission to accomplish and we were simply making strategic decisions on how to best accomplish it. Heck of a game of "battle-ship", don't you agree? I decided that "no emotion" was better than "bad emotion". Now, at this instant, there was no ignoring it, that whole "calm, strategic plan" went straight to hell. It was time. He, being Dr. Montalban, had already come in to "mark" me. I remember clearly starting to wonder silently if I'm not just slightly crazy for not being hysterical. Let's face it. This doctor is using some marker, which is a lovely shade of purple, to mark where he is going to cut me open and tell me … tell me?

Tell me to go home, hug Jim and go on with me life.

Vivid

I can replay the next hour and half over in my mind and not skip a beat. I can even see the sweat on the Drs.' Brow, and there was a lot, honey. Kind of makes you wonder why you are not sweating. I am laying in the operating room Filled with doctors, nurses, neonatal staff, blah, blah, blah. Let's just say, not as many people as a Prince concert, but more than a "frat" party. I have this curtain at the base of my neck, preventing me from seeing the work that he is doing. Yet, because I am fully awake, I can hear the sound of the scalpel, the suctioning out of my blood from the skin that had been cut open. I feel pain. So much pain, for the love of God, help me.

One of the nurses is at the base of my head. How wonderful she is. Caressing my hair. Talking about everything, anything. Like when you are stuck in the elevator on a long ride up, and you feel you have to say something. Yet, this was not as awkward as the stinky guy in the elevator. She seemed to be a nice lady, someone that would be a nice friend, if we had met under different situations, you know. I was so glad to have her there. "I can feel it, I can feel it," I would say to her, and Ricardo and they would give me another shot.

Then the "physical" pain would leave, but only for a short time it seemed, and the whole process would repeat itself. This went on, it seemed like forever, but wait, it gets worse. Then at last I hear the words everyone in the room was desperately hoping to hear.

"This isn't cancer. I can tell this isn't cancer. Looks like you're a lucky woman, Robin!" I could tell he was putting the mass in a container that a nurse was holding. I looked up at the nurse that had comforted me threw it all. We must have been acting as mirrors.

Her smile was just as large and as beautifully wide as mine must have been. Her eyes said, "I'm so happy for you." **I was in heaven!** They were cleaning me up, unhooking all the surgical apparatus from my body, and me? I was in heaven. Closing my eyes in peace, I thought to myself. Thoughts of pure, simple, innocent thankfulness and new babies came into mind. I turned my head to the side and saw doc on the phone. That's weird, I remember thinking. Who the heck would you be calling after you just performed surgery and gave some woman the best news of her life. Then it hit me. He's a doctor, stupid. He's probably calling to see if he can still grab that tee time. I mean c'mon he turns out a couple surgeries before lunch. I soon found out whom it was he was really talking to. The lab is a place I have since learned to accept for it's painfully, slow pace, due to their very accurate, yet usually, not welcomed news.

I looked over again. I looked dead into his eyes with the face of sheer bliss to thank him. I formed my hands to give him two "thumbs up". He looked at me, paused for just an instant, and gave me two "thumbs down". That's how I knew. I knew. That's how I was told I had cancer. I could feel the silent tear stream down my cheek. It burned. His walk over to me seemed to be in slow motion. His words cut me sharper than any scalpel ever could. "Let me go get your husband Robin" … and then it came. I looked up at the nurse … she was crying. The room was so hot,

God, it was hot in there. The emotional faucet that I had cranked closed so very tight turned on and I let go. I lost it. Crying so hard my body was almost convulsing. I couldn't stop. Then I noticed the whole room was filled with tears. People I didn't even know felt my pain. Caressing my stomach. My baby, oh God, my daughter, Oh God, Jim. I was so very sorry for him.

Oh God … help us.

I don't remember getting to see Jim. Whether he came to see me, or they moved me to a different room. My mind just cuts to when I saw him.

There weren't any words. We were somehow instantaneously beyond that. We spoke more in those moments in recovery, without saying a word, than one could ever imagine. There was a silence that was more meaningful than we ever had with words before, or ever will again. Two hearts, silently breaking for each other, silently breaking for us. Breaking for our children, born and unborn … Oh God … help us.

I remember the drive home as long. I looked out the window at farms and fields I must have seen a thousand times before. And yet they looked so different. Peaceful. Now, you know I'm stressed if Michigan is starting to look good to me. When we got home, I remember tripping out on the fact he was opening the door to our first home. I looked up to the knocker. "The Dyes-Established in 1996" It was a gift from a girlfriend, Dana McDonald, who sold us the house. That was hard. It was scary too because I knew once we were inside the door there wasn't going to be any distractions. Just Jim and I were, alone, with cancer. I lay down on our bed and cry. I decided that I would give myself that. I would lay for a while on our bed, with Jim and fall apart. Then, I would be strong. I had to be. For

Jim, who had just lost his mother, for my daughter who would look to me for assurance, for my unborn child, for my friends who were terrified, and, for myself. If I could just stay factual about this whole thing and go through the steps, it will all be over. I justified it, as stupid as it sounds, like a roller coaster ride. I hate em. In fact they terrify the crap out of me. But somehow, every summer at the amusement parks I find myself in the seat, entrusting my life to some high school kid making 6 bucks an hour for a summer job, and I pace myself through it. For the forty-five minutes I wait in line, I watch the ride over and over again. Pacing the movements, counting the seconds between turns and upside down twists of the track and so when I get in the seat. I close my eyes and just mentally go through the ride counting out the turns and spins I memorized in my head until it's over and I'm back at the beginning. That's how I could handle this. We'll go and find out the steps, I'll pace it out, and just close my eyes and go through it. Yeah … that'll work.

Then reality creeps in and you start feeling the fear … the pain … the overwhelming sense that your going to die. It was a mental battle in me that I've never experienced before, and hope I never do again. The battle to convince myself I was going to live.

Who the hell gave it the right to come into my life? Then I decided, right then and there … enough. I got really, really pissed off. And all I could think about was that I wasn't gong down like this. I refuse to die. I absolutely refuse to let cancer take me out. I mean, who the hell gave it the right to come into my life? Along with that, I remember being grateful that of all the girls in my family that could have found out they had cancer today, that it was I. Maybe, God allowed this to happen to me because he thought I could handle it. Handle it. Handle it? I don't want to handle it.

I want to put it on the counter and smash its' bloody face in with a iron cast skillet, scrap up the remains and put it in the trash and get it the hell out of my home. But there isn't anyone to take it out on. No one is responsible. That, I think, is the worst part. If any person had brought this type of agony upon you, or your family, If you knew who had caused the pain you see deep in your husbands eyes, the fear that he won't admit to ... you would beat them uncontrollably with every fiber of your body and soul. You would then drink their blood. ('Ole Latin saying) Taking full gratification in their slow agony. But there's no one. This unseen bastard has done this ... and you have no retaliation.

But there is retaliation ... it's called, survival.

Survive. That's what I set out to do. That's why I write this book.

So that when another person, or the loved one of that person, finds that they have a similar, or what seems to be the "God forsaken" situation of life, that they may look at my survival, my conquer, against all the odds, lab results and doctors prognosis, and walk away with the crystal clear conviction that if I can do it; me, a "Nobody, from Nowhere" just the "girl from down the street, that, with God, so can they. Or, you're damned sure going to give it your all. With determination and a smile. Don't just "survive", "Conquer". Have, and take or grab some, courage.

John17: 6 In this world you will have trouble. But take heart I have overcome the world.

The Hunt:

The hunt is on! Should it be this doctor, or that one? It is pretty much a "crapshoot" on" the hunt". What are you hunting for? You hunt for one doctor, any doctor, to be a "good little boy" and tell you there's been some crazy mix up … their "extremely sorry for the scare", "never happened before in the history of" … blah, blah, blah. This was not to be. We were told everything from "we have to take the baby", to "you've got limited time due to the aggressive nature and size" blah, blah, blah and then there's every other doctors' diagnosis; and then, there's "Jo-Jo". Blessing.

Jo-Jo~(Dr. Joseph Kingsbury)

They talk about patients falling in love with their doctor/with a savior syndrome. Honey, you have no idea. Nor will I give you one in detail now. Let me say he has all the qualities a Latin woman like me adores.

Intelligence, skill, beyond handsome, successful in his field, and fatherhood, and loves the "blues and jazz", oh and did I mention … he saved, not just my life, but also my unborn Childs'?

"Jo Jo" came as a "hidden" blessing. Friend of a friend, knows this doctor they remolded for, "Hell of a good doctor, think you should see him", sort of non-chalent deal the way Tamara put it or so I thought at the time. I remember, "The Call" was placed, he cancelled his golf, and then I remember hearing the voice like it was in slow motion, like the voice of the teacher on Charlie Brown … "I know its short notice but can you come in tomorrow?" Meeting Dr. Jo in his office at Genesis Hospital turned out to be the first, clear turning point towards the light at the end of the rainbow. The first day of the rest of my life happened that day. I realized much later how very close I was to losing that/my life, and my child. Besides I always thought my savior would be all dressed in black, like "Zorro". I didn't expect the whole hospital scrubs thing. Especially, in that tacky shade of "barf" green he had. That was so unacceptable, *really*.

"Can you keep me alive?

Can you promise me, WE won't die? Tell me, for all that is right with the world. Tell me … tell me … there is a God.…"! Tell me Jo, that you are as good as they say.

Tell me … tell me … tell me. Kind of like that whole "Sam Kineson" act … Say it … Say it … Ugh. Say it …

The words," those" words, they didn't come from him. "Reaction"? His eyes … they said, and what he spoke, was compassion, empathy, confidence, most importantly, **honesty.**

"Robin, I don't know, I am going to try like hell though. We just don't know. We don't know if you're going to make it. But Robin, we are going to try like hell"

To remember; verbatim, thank you, his words, his look, his eyes, at "that" moment, spawns many emotions now. I do remember being so pleased he has a pleasant personality, the guy "next door" type of demeanor. Him smiling with his eyes, at my sad, nervous attempts at humor. That whole uncomfortable elevator ride with me attempted to talk. Yep, that was Robin Renee.

I realize now with all the non~welcomed experience I have with Doctors' real limitations. Their "only human" skill becomes apparent. How unfair of me it was to ask those questions.

The "strategic plan was set.

Dr. Kingsbury and his "Plan To Fight"

Steroids for the babies' lungs
Stay calm/act normal for the baby's sake
Keep testing for the steroids to work.
Wait
Act normal
Stay calm
Be cool, man. Wait to put all this behind us, and live like I did. Stay calm, act normal and be cool. This shouldn't be a problem, I am the "cool, funny one; remember? I am in control. Not, of this *shit* disease. I am in control of my demeanor. My "mind set". I will be strong. My father says, and I completely agree, "No-one can control if there is a smile on your face or not, but *you*. It may happen ... but how you *"let"* it affect you and your day, and your smile? That is *entirely up to you.* Bigger picture you ask? I am pretty sure, I don't "know", because he doesn't phone or fax me personally, I do think Jesus knew "all along" how His story on earth would end. Don't you?

You didn't see Him with the whole "Poor pitiful me" deal. This is what I call the "EEYORE" disease. Well, I have cancer, not the "Eeyore" syndrome. Oh, and did I mention ... I am going to live? I don't give a crap what anyone else on this planet says or what he or she really thinks. What came next?

Honestly I can't spread the "wait" out for you with any full/clear detail .I do remember substantial moments. I will touch on those for you're reading pleasure. It was not the "minutes", but the memories are important. I pray this for you too.

Luke12: 2,5.Who of you by worrying can add a single hour to his life? Since you cannot do this very little thing, why do you worry about the rest?

CHEMO-*Therapy*

I have no idea what or how this whole part of the puzzle lays out, really. Again, I rely on memories, rather than moments. I was just telling friends about this "flash" the other day. It all started when the "chemo" doc comes in my "birthing room" at the hospital. One morning after they took "Faith", my beautiful daughter, out of my diseased body. "How important, Robin, is it that you don't lose your hair?" This question will burn in the memory bank forever. Odd, I thought. He looks like a relatively intelligent guy, hospital scrubs and all, you know I adore that barf green shade, does he know, I mean, has he looked at the chart? Hello … stupid man. They just cut my stomach wide open, took out my child early, you know, the one in the bassinette, right there.

Oh yeah, and did you **see** in the chart? They just cut my breast off. They cut the "perky" one off, thank you. The right one, the one that would help me win any dispute that intelligence, or common sense, wouldn't? HELLO!! You piece of dog crap! Is this your attempt at humor? Are you high? Are you now, or when you looked at the chart? I remember getting so violently upset, instantly, but inside. Now that I look back, he wasn't the one to take it out on, anyways. There isn't anyone. But, be there no mistake. I am thankful for my dad teaching me to control of my own, at times, brutal, temper. I remember controlling my temper a lot. I believe, looking back, that it was the smart, compassionate, and respectful, even if it was respecting my own honor, not theirs, thing to do.

James 1:19 My dear brothers, take note of this: Everyone should be quick to listen, slow to speak and slow to become angry, for mans' anger does not bring about the righteous life God desires.

Picking out the boob

If given the right circumstances … like, um alcohol, good friends, or a microphone; this is, hysterical. If you're a man … imagine. Picking out your cock. Delightful! Really. Really the bonus package, or that's what you'd pick out, anyways. Do I miss my breasts? YES. I never, however regret the choice I made. I believe you always have a choice. No matter what, there is a choice. Child or tit was the choice. Hum … let's weigh that one, for just a moment. I have found, and this maybe, just me, that any part of your body, is just that … a part. Given the choice I had, I kiss my daughter, Faith, the true love of my life, as both my daughters are, everyday. Shit, I digress again. Can you imagine how much easier talking would be for me over writing? It's painful really. The boob. Defiant, as I am, to my core, this poor woman who had the unfortunate luck to be working that day was in tears, I think from laughing, when I left. I will never "Know". Like a shy child, when I'm uncomfortable, for whatever reason, I act, um, flamboyant. A friend once told me I was overwhelming. Well, when I'm uncomfortable, honey, they never have a chance to meet "me". Not the real me anyways. I'm not going to give them the chance to see how venerable, scared and sad I am. Nope. Not going to happen.

Who or what gives people the honor of knowing the real you? Only you do. You determined what you choose to let people know or see about you. I did give a heck of a stand up comedian act walking into their store. Smile and charm. I told the story how my mother, Carolyn, had just donated a boob, to breast cancer. She, being strong willed as well, decided a "nerf" football, cut just right, felt more natural. This of course, until she leaned over a centerpiece, and found out, quite rudely, that they are not, however, flames resistant.

She phoned almost in tears saying "I just caught my boob on fire". I guess you had to be there. Kind of like the boob store.

It's like a plethora of breasts. Every shape, every size/color, if you can name it, oh, they've got it. If I was a perverted lesbian, that would be my new hangout. A beer, and I'd be set. Boob, in box, I told myself I was well on the way to recovery. I also determined I could do the ice cream on the way home because measuring how much the boob weighed I just lost 5 lbs. I was due. I do not think; one should, over think. It is over rated. Just give it up to God.

Psalm55: 22 Cast your cares on the Lord and he will sustain you; he will never let the righteous fall.

The eyelash

When I look at those times, I remember certain odd or funny times, too. Could you imagine for one second, refusing not to put mascara on that one little eyelash you have left? That would again be me. It was to be against all doctor or family and friends counsel. I absolutely refused to put that pink tube of great lash mascara down or to throw it out. I saw it as the last string of femininity I had left. Cancer had taken my hair, taken my breasts, taken my eyebrows, skin color and overall feeling of health. There was no way I was going to donate the mascara. No way. It somehow gave me a sense of normalcy putting it on. Is it normal to get pink eye? No. It was a barter or trade I agreed to. I have to tell you, that one little lash was looking mighty curly and long. No clumps or black rub off on the skin. It is amazing how it works when you focus and do it right. The point you ask? The message to take is it does not matter if it is putting on a chicken suit, going down your main street and barking like a dog, if it gives you comfort in your hours of discomfort, whether they are physical or mental, do it. Make sure not to hurt anyone else though. If taking out the people in line somewhere is what you are thinking ... go home, and think again.

The Sick Days

There were plenty of days when I felt like I had a serious hangover in my stomach. My head couldn't think, and I thank God Jim was there to take care of Faith and friends brought over the delightfully creative casseroles (a lot of them; who knew, that casseroles are so diverse?) I simply couldn't take care of myself on some days, let alone our house, or our bran new baby. Thankfully, looking back, those days were few and I pray that anyone who may be enduring the same trial, his or her days of grieving or aching are few too. The days spent enjoying life and Faith and Felizia were more prevalent. I was; and am, determined to remind myself that there are a lot of reasons to live, and I hold on to them with a death grip (pardon the term) during that time and still do. I also, and I recommend it to you, laughed ALOT. When I only had one little black curly eyelash left … I had to laugh at trying to put mascara on it. What's the point, really? I gave myself eye infections because I refused to listen to men, doctors, or anyone that tried to tell me to give it up. Me? Never! There is a saying that one can't see the trees despite the forest. Honey, I made sure to see every leaf. Every groove in the trunk, smelt every budding, admired every color change. To say that "dieing" makes you aware of "living". That is an understatement.

It is good, but it brings a sense of sadness only you; and the depths of your spirit, with Gods' help can shake or endure. This is where the point of Testament lies. You, just like us all, and I did, must; absolutely must, use your spirit, self determination and the will and inner strength Jehovah gave you to get thru whatever you must, with His help. Otherwise you can; and probably will, get sucked into an even worse disease ... the Eeyore one. Just say no! Say no to anyone, no matter the title, or anything, that tries to tell you to give up! Be strong, and remember you can!

Whatever the question, the answer is yes, you can. Believe it. Believe it with all your heart and the spirit God gave you. He believes in you. Why shouldn't you?

Memories~

Cheryl Peacock.

My friend now, was my boss/friend then. The one I called and said I wouldn't be returning from the doctors' appointment that day. I was in her office, which was right behind my desk. Everyone thinks it was because we were friends. I think not. I think it was a "love/hate relationship from the jump. "They were watching me ... the bastards. I didn't often or really ever follow proper procedures" that burned them. I was, however, always blowing radio sales goals out of the water or at least holding my own. That burned them too. That means they have to leave me alone. I personally, ate that crap up☺

But, I digress. In the office, which was too small, in relation to her importance to the company, I thought. In the office, trying to be cool controlled funny one ... Going over goals and potential new business leads. I remember letting Cheryl's eyes of empathy hit my "I've got a brutal secret" ones, and letting myself crack for the first moment since "Jo Jo's" strategic office meeting.

I broke down, and if she wanted to see the emotions I was hiding. Honey, she got the "bonus" family package ... super sized package. I remember saying, almost begging clear as ice, "I don't want to die, Cheryl. *It isn't in my planner.*

*I'm too young and cute to die. I just don't want to die now. **Not now, not like this.**"* Just picture that scene from the "Titanic" ... *they* copycatted. Honey, I did the first rendition and Cheryl will testify to the same. You know, once I pay her back that twenty, she will be good for whatever ☺

Then, of course, it was back to the cool, calm, funny, or trying to be funny me. I had had absolutely enough of that. The whining, poor pitiful me "Eeyore" crap just was not my M.O. I was not going to make it my m.o., either. Not over cancer. It was not going to take that too!

Friends

The one event that will undoubtedly happen, no matter who you are, no matter what the "trauma", is well, a "drama" in itself. Be prepared. There is no way to prepare. The whole friends issue. I was pleasantly surprised, and yet, violently, stupidly, disappointed. It's unavoidable, really. Kindhearted people that you didn't even put in your mental roster of friends will be there in your hours of need w/whatever they can do. Dinners for your family, watching the kids, (you know, when the barf sessions are on overdrive) or anything you may need help with. Believe me; bud, after going through a couple traumas myself, you going to need a lot of help. It is necessary, whether you want it or not.

It is all stemming from good intentions. It is the people you think are friends, ah, now see, that's the jacked part. I had a so-called friend, that once the hair was gone, even the eyebrows, the boobs were gone, and the skin was looking like a dress rehearsal for "Fright Night" she without any hesitation, *bailed out*. Not to be seen for a long time. I, after smacking myself upside the head for being so stupid that I was still shocked at peoples' behavior, gave up with trying to track her down. She did show up at my door step almost 1 ½ years later and say she "just couldn't deal with seeing me like that", Hello … should I feel something for you here?

Because I really don't mind telling you actually I got to tell you, I would tell you, I feel nothing for you. Should I feel guilty that the sights of my dying body made you feel uneasy? Are you a self-absorbed person now, or were you then? All I can say is the moments that followed after I opened the door; well, they weren't pretty. Actually, down right ugly. They were ugly for her maybe. Not me.

To me, the death of our supposed friendship happened when she bailed on me. The mourning process for that supposed friendship had already occurred. Of course, I had to work it in around the whole falling apart inside for my own life … you know.

We all have our priorities, baby. I have been very blessed with people I love, and those that love me. I have now, and for a long time have had, good, true friends. Going through a "Trauma" sucks. Period. But I certainly saw peoples' true heart, this at times was a blessing, at others a detriment. You should cherish the blessings for they may be rare. Forget the other moments. I have tried to share with you memories of smiles, and laughter. Tried, being the key word. Don't think for one moment that the crap wasn't there. It was.

"Was" In saying "was", meaning they were in the past. I got through it. Will you? I have no way of knowing. Neither do you, or any doctor, friend, or counselor. Only God does, and He's not big on faxes and phone call updates. BUT you can ask Him.

I believe, if you convince your mind that you will; your heart, and your body may follow. It will definitely have a better chance. Remember that whole choice deal? You've got one! No matter what! Love, yourself, enough not to let someone, no matter what their official title is, try to make you believe you don't have that choice. Even if, you are just waiting for the last heroin shot, to let you slip off into "never, never" land, it is how you carry yourself there that may determine how your flight is. It may even determine it's final destination too☺ People I know say that it is easy for me to speak this way, now, that I have conquered cancer. Honey, I was speaking this way when I was three. Times, to my own detriment. It is easy to confuse my style with that of one being pompous. I spoke this way, and had a positive attitude, long before "terminal" cancer. Is it really important, what the battle is against? I think not. Kick its butt! Kick it, to the point it wouldn't dare think of messing with you again or any longer.

You are, you. Beautiful person. You wouldn't give up your space in line at a coffee café, waiting for that "Moose Munch Mocha". Don't dare … give up on you. U.B.U. You're fantastic. Your scars, disease, memories, family, friends, addictions, convictions, body, mind, heart, soul, beliefs, faith, opinions and everything else that is a piece of your puzzle; make up, you. You are a beautiful human being. Remember that!

If God made us in His image, and I know he did, He must have been damned fine, 'because you're not bad yourself.

Well, at least I know, I'm not.

I had gone, after all of these, trails, tribulations, lessons and moments of enlightenment, on vacation to Miami. I and we, being Faith and I had made it to the "special safe" time of five years. Just to be safe, we waited for the sixth year. The whole family met. I mean, the whole family. There was everyone except my sister Dawn Michelle' and my brother Kenneth Marshall's' family, which was a loss that we'll never be able to undo. There was swimming in the ocean, playing at the beach, banana boat rides, tanning and drinks mixed with pizza, movies and tent making time with all the kids. I absolutely was on top of the world. It was to be the best holiday ever. Was it? I imagine you'll have to read Testament II to judge for yourself.

Off with the wig!

One of the other memories that stand out is the day I took off the wig. I had been very selective when I purchased it, and it was, in my opinion, a damned good one. The average person would have, could have, never known it was a wig. When I went back to work at the radio station most of my co-workers had no idea I had lost my hair. I do not believe they had any idea I had been fighting so hard to stay alive, either. I am, and will be forever grateful of that. It enabled me to hold my head up, laugh and try to go about the workday like a "normal" person.

We were all in our staff meeting in the conference room, the meeting was over and Cheryl addressed everyone and said I had something to share. This is another memory that is so clear I can tell you what everyone was wearing, the color of their lipstick, and the smell of each ones perfume. All eyes were on me, with that "Well, what ya got?" look. I stated this, "Some one you are aware of how sick I have been with my struggle with cancer, some not. I have decided that I no longer wish to put on this charade of having hair, when I don't. Please don't be scared, but I wanted to share with you guys first ..." I pulled off the wig, sat and looked. I looked them back right in the eyes. I saw; I saw, warmth. I saw an overwhelming feeling of strength and support that surprised even me. There were comments like, "you look great, Robin" to "it's like our own Sinead O'Connor" to "I had no idea" to "Can I touch?". When it was done, I felt an immense feeling of strength. I felt strength from them, strength from Cheryl, strength from myself. It was the right time and the right decision. Besides I was getting hot under that thing. Time to cool off and cool down. You must decide these times by yourself.

No one can tell you it's time. It is, a very personal decision, that you cannot go back on or change your mind. Be strong and He will, too.

GOD wants spiritual fruit, not religious nuts.

Dear God, it's me, I have a problem.

There is no key to happiness. The door is always open.

Silence is often misinterpreted, but never misquoted.

Do the math and count your blessings.

Faith gives the ability not to panic.

Laugh every day, it is jogging for the soul.

If you worry, you did not pray. If you pray, do not worry.

As a child of God, praying is like calling home.

Blessed are the flexible, for they will not be bent out of shape.

The most important thing in a home, are the people in it.

If you are tangled in problems, be still, so God can untangle you.

A grudge is a heavy thing to carry,

He who dies with the most possessions, in the end, is still dead.

We won't remember the days, just the moments.

~ Reflect ~

Corinthians 8:1 . We know we all possess knowledge. Knowledge puffs up but love builds up. The man who thinks he knows something does not yet know, as he ought to know.

Matthew 7:1,2. Do not judge, or you too will be judged. For in the same way you judge others, you will be judged, and with the measure you use, it will be measured to you.

Luke12: 2,5.Who of you by worrying can add a single hour to his life? Since you cannot do this very little thing, why do you worry about the rest?

Deuteronomy 26:18.And the Lord has declared this day, that you are His people, His treasured possession as he promised,

Galatians 6:4.Each one should test his own actions. Then he can take pride in himself without comparing himself to somebody else, for each one should carry his own load.

Ezekiel 22:14.Will your courage endure or your hands be strong the day I deal with you? I the Lord have spoken, and I will do it.

Matthew 6:5 "And when you pray, do not be like the hypocrites, for they love to pray standing in synagogues and on the street corners to be seen by men. I tell you the truth; they have received their reward in full. But when you pray, go into your room, close the door, and pray to your Father, who is unseen. Then your Father, who sees what is done in secret, will reward you. And when you pray, do not keep on babbling like pagans, for they think they will be heard because of their many words. Do not be like them, for your Father knows what you need, before you ask him".

James 1:19 My dear brothers, take note of this: Everyone should be quick to listen, slow to speak and slow to become angry, for man's anger does not bring about the righteous life God desires.

John17: 6. In this world you will have trouble. But take heart I have overcome the world.

Psalm55: 22 Cast your cares on the Lord and he will sustain you; he will never let the righteous fall.

Final Thought~

IT IS OKAY TO SIT ON YOUR PITY POT EVERY ONCE IN
AWHIEL, JUST REMEMBER TO FLUSH WHEN DONE.

May you be aware that, Jehovah has blessed you all, *already!*

978-0-595-40820-7
0-595-40820-6

www.ingramcontent.com/pod-product-compliance
Lightning Source LLC
Chambersburg PA
CBHW050336290526
45785CB00006B/2519